Easing into the Bhagavad Gita
and Patanjali's Yoga Sutras

by

Kimberly Beyer-Nelson, MA, CHHC, CYTh, RM

Cover design by Kathy Haug

You can contact Kathy for cover design ideas at:

http://ferncreekassociates.com/

To all my teachers,

from the ones who walk on two feet,

to the stillest of stones

and all the life of spirit in between--

I bow to thee palm to palm.

Introduction

When new students walk into a Hatha Yoga class, the chances are they won't know much about texts like the *Bhagavad Gita* or *Patanjali's Yoga Sutras*. But the teacher who only gives physical postures and breath-work and meditation is offering the smallest sliver of the richness of India's spiritual technologies. And why do I use that word, *technologies*, very consciously? Because I will be the first to argue that any of the great Yogas may be used as a spiritual tool that can be adapted to any religious or spiritual tradition. It is perfectly right and good to be a Buddhist Yogi or a Christian or Jewish Yogi for example. Most the yogas make provision for *your* ideal, your understanding of God or ultimate reality. The divine is big enough to hold all conceptualizations.

At some point, there will be a few students who want to know more than what the physical practice hints at. They will want to understand the philosophy, the intent behind the tool of Hatha and other Yoga. The very stillness and mindfulness of their work eventually calls up questions like:

1. What is the nature of the divine and how do I participate in it?

2. How do I still the noise of my mind?

3. What is this thing called karma? Dharma? Samadhi?

4. How do I take this peace I feel in my yoga class off the mat and into the world?

5. Do relationships and families make following a spiritual path impossible or at least very difficult? Or can they be the very ground of practice?

6. AND SO ON!

And that is the precise moment when having at least a rudimentary understanding of these beautiful and sometimes difficult ancient texts will elevate you from a technical teacher to a way-shower, a light-bringer, for the human soul. You can open a door for someone into a wider worldview. And to tell the truth, spiritual inquiry is what really guides most of us to a yoga class, even if we aren't consciously aware of that fact. Honest practitioners of Hatha Yoga are not so much concerned about whether or not they look good in lycra, but rather, seek to experience an inkling of how freedom and devotion *feels*. So this little book will attempt to sketch you a first map, if you will, of two of the best-known spiritual texts of India. You may find your own fires of interest kindled and you may want to dig more deeply into why these ancient works continue to speak to human beings in this place and age. If so, you will find it is a journey well worth taking.

You'll find I've included lots of questions for group discussion, too, because we don't really "feel" a spiritual text until it breathes within our own skins and dances with our own life experiences. I sketch, in other words, but you? You have the paints and crayons and magic markers of your personal experience and expression that will make this all come to life.

The Bhagavad Gita: 10 Points to Ponder

Hundreds of translations.

Thousands of years of commentaries.

Inspiration for music, film, paintings, theater,

philosophical inquiry.

But

what does it offer us,

the teachers and students of Hatha Yoga

today?

*B*efore you sit down to work with these essays and questions, find a copy of the Bhagavad Gita you resonate with. My favorite is actually one that isn't particularly scholarly but the language is poetic, alive, even passionate. Be willing to thumb through a number of them at your favorite bookstore or on-line. It's a bit like buying clothes—find the color and fit that is right for you. Then actually read it! The Gita is rather short, and in a day or two you can breeze through it, hearing the poetry, gathering impressions, maybe just basking in the glorious 10th and 11th chapters that might comprise the most incredible song about God ever put to pen and paper.

As you begin, keep in mind this is a slice of history you are holding as well. The Gita was written sometime between 500 BCE to 200 CE, although parts of its thought may have existed in spoken form for much longer, making its true dating much more difficult. Part of the huge *Mahabharata*, one of the great epic poems of India that is about seven times the size of the *Iliad* and *Odyssey* combined, the entire teaching of the Gita (all 700ish lines of verse) takes place on a battlefield, alongside a chariot poised between two great armies.

If you can bring this kind of immediacy to your reading, really feeling the pressures shaping the conversation between Arjuna, the royal archer and Krishna the charioteer (and an *avatar* of God), the text will begin to come alive for you. And when you make the cognitive jump—that we all must battle the voices within us, voices that originate not just with our closest family members but from our society at large, when the field of battle becomes the field within your own mind and heart, you will have taken one more step into *why* this text continues to be translated and commented upon even in this age of space-flight and cell phones and nano-technology.

You could spend a lifetime with this text—memorizing it, chanting it, watching your own life to see where it applies. But let's say you just have a weekend to first shake its hand. What ten things would really stand out in this text? What ten points could you take to heart and really ponder and bring to your work on and off the Hatha Yoga mat?

What follows is "My Top Ten Important Ideas from the Bhagavad Gita." (After you've read the Gita a few times, you may have a totally different list. But all journeys begin at some point. I'm pleased we'll step out together from here, even if your own path branches off in the future. Indeed, it should.)

The Top Ten Important Ideas from the Bhagavad Gita

1. No measure of spiritual devotion or practice is ever wasted.

2. The unity of the organs of perception, the perceiver and the perceived (or, in other words, the known, the knower and knowing are all one).

3. Performing your own dharma is critical in life.

4. Divine revelation and experience is not just given to the professional religious among us.

5. For the many personalities of people, there is a yoga (path to union with the divine) that is suitable for them.

6. We have a right to our actions, but not to the fruits of our actions. Those belong only to God.

7. The sage established in wisdom is free of desires, content, untroubled by fortune or misfortune, free of craving, fear, anger, and aversion, focused wholly on God.

8. The person who thinks they kill or that they can be killed is dwelling in ignorance.

9. Radical monotheism: God is both immanent and transcendent, both huge and small, both inner and outer.

10. All living things must act; even God.

1. *No measure of spiritual devotion or practice is ever wasted.*

One of the most poignant questions Arjuna asks Krishna is this: "If I follow this path of union through action, meditation or knowledge, but then I fall away from it, will all my work be lost?" This is so very human of Arjuna; he is assuming that there are concrete beginnings and endings; that he is part of a world of acquisition and stolen moments and objects; that he is a finite creature in a finite world. But Krishna is quick to tell him that no measure of spiritual devotion is ever wasted. Not one meditation practice, not one pure action, not one bowed knee of awe and praise is ever lost. It is a jewel in the heart, outside of the vagaries of time and place.

But how can this be?

It is important to keep in mind there is no scorekeeper in this philosophy. And while karma, cause and effect, make for effective referees if we actually learn from their calls, the *actions* we take rest in our own hands. Any movement that reconnects us to the idea of "tat tvam asi" (Thou Art That) is never lost because time and the divine don't work in a linear fashion. Any small crack that allows the light of God to shine through cannot be plugged up because it is a taste of what we truly are. "For all beings, Joy is inevitable," says Yudhisthira (Arjuna's older brother and heir to the throne). And for all beings, waking up to our participation in and continuance with the divine is also inevitable.

Even if (and it will) take many lifetimes.

How still the branches bared to cold,

how hard the ground, nearly gray with decay and frost,

how weathered, the old barn door, squeaking as it opens.

But a warm nose comes to my hand, nostrils flaring steamy breath

hooves shuffle on hard-packed earth, impatient.

See!

Life echoes here,

This great-grandchild of my first horse,

And I see through her soft brown eye,

The cascade of her lineage,

Back to the time when fire burst out in the total darkness,

"Let there be light! And Horses! For I AM!"

And in her eye,

See my own, reflected.

KBN 2013

Questions to Ponder:

1. How does this point differ from the message other religious scriptures often imply? In what ways is it similar?

2. How do you show your devotion to the divine in your life? How important is this to your own sense of well-being? Explain.

3. Why is this an important message for Arjuna to receive? Is it an important message for you to hear? Why or why not?

4. How can you convey the idea of devotion to your Hatha Yoga students in a way that honors their various spiritual paths?

5. Is there a shadow side to religious/spiritual devotion? What might that be?

2. The unity of the organs of perception, the perceiver and the perceived (or, in other words, the known, the knower and knowing are all one).

OK, now don't throw the e-reader or book across the room. This concept is not as difficult as it sounds. Let's break it down slowly.

First the *organs of perception* are all your senses—eye, ear, nose, mouth/tongue, nerve-endings. But an eyeball sitting on a kitchen counter isn't capable of seeing, nor can an ear, by itself, hear anything at all, let alone identify and *name* what it is hearing. What lies behind the senses of perception? The brain, and more importantly, consciousness.

The *perceiver* is you, at first glance. "I see. I feel. I taste." But again, *who are you*? This, by the way, could be the only question you need to use to "wake up" to Reality. Keep asking yourself "who am I?" over and over again, writing down a different answer each time. Now look carefully at the list. Are you simply your roles, relationships, age, gender, etc? Or is there something ineffable that is ultimately you? And what relationship does that quality of self share with the divine? Or is it more than a sharing? Again, if you keep at this practice, you will eventually come to the conclusion that the base of the perceiver is consciousness, pure and undiluted.

And the perceived? That is what the eye, ear, nose, mouth/tongue and nerves *respond to*. But again, even if you are able to say, see a candle, there is something within you that is the root, the base, used to identify the object. You may find yourself comparing it to other candles, experience memories of lighting other candles, etc. Even if you really can see just this candle, just this present moment object, what is doing that experiencing? Consciousness. Yes.

So, consciousness is the name for the union of the organs of perception, the perceiver and the perceived. And what is consciousness? Ah…now you are at the door to a much wider world, and Krishna is smiling at you with an open hand.

A hand I dipped in the restless sea,

Sea, a clamshell echoed back to me,

Me, and yet more than this body,

Body, swelling with breath,

Breath tickling mind,

Mind falling into intuition,

Intuition into joy,

Joy at my hand dancing, dallying with the cold, gray sea.

KBN 2013

Questions to Ponder:

1. Describe, in concrete terms, the perceiver, the perceived and perception in a way you could share with your yoga students.

2. What are the life ramifications of this philosophy? In other words, if you lived your life from this perspective, how would you view education? Shopping? Your partner? God?

3. What other religious traditions teach this idea? Can you give an example?

4. How does this idea change the way you might respond to:

    a. An angry person?

    b. A pile of doggie-doo in your yard?

    c. Someone you feel is more powerful or knowledgeable than you?

    d. A creative impulse?

5. In what ways does this philosophy fly in the face of your own cultural upbringing?

6. How might a scientist respond to this idea?

3. *Performing your own dharma is critical in life.*

The word dharma is a slippery one. Here, it might include the tastes of role, duty, action, and life-course all mixed together. At first blush, this might be considered one of those common sense kinds of sayings. "Of course I "do" my own dharma. How could I not?"

But sometimes it's not that easy. I spent about thirty years of my life trying to live up to what I thought other people wanted me to do; and the deepest part of myself kept rebelling so I ended up in a kind of stuck place, not going forward, not living my own life, either. It may be a grace for many of us that we begin to live our dharma more easily as we age.

I remember a story from when I was an undergraduate. A professor led a deep imagination session with his class in which the students essentially pictured themselves at their own deathbeds. They were instructed to ask that dying self what they should be doing with their lives, right now, in the present. Afterward, one young man was really agitated by the exercise. His parents and grandparents were lawyers, and he was expected to follow in their footsteps. He loved photography, but "knew" that he could never make a life for himself doing what he loved. He stormed into the professor's office and told him in no uncertain terms that his dying self had been wrong; he was going to be a lawyer, not a photographer. The professor shrugged, calmed him down and school broke for the summer later that week.

As school started up again in the fall, the young man was once again in the professor's office—with a camera around his neck, and full of light. He went on to do incredible photojournalism work for major magazines. There are many lawyers, but he gave the world a unique gift with his photography. It was his dharma to do so.

Now, not all of us will have such powerful stories to tell. Stories like this are bigger than life, almost parables. And certainly in Arjuna's case, Krishna is trying to show him that his dharma isn't sweet, creative or aesthetically pleasing particularly. It's going to be tedious, bloody, filled with pain. But it is *his* path, the very fiber of his being, and to vary from it will send a ripple out into the world, like a stone dropped into a pond creates a vacuum that, for a moment, pulls the rest of the water down and in.

We might kick at our dharma, as Arjuna certainly does But here, the Gita is particularly medicinal—for Krishna tells Arjuna, "These men you see arrayed before you, uncles, grandfathers, cousins? Do you think they can be killed? Do you think that you are the one doing the killing? That is ignorance." Remember the previous point: "the organs of perception, the perceiver and the perceived are one." Who kills on this field? Who dies? If God is the very ground of reality, then all of this is play. God is the doer, not the constructed ego.

This is not an injunction to do whatever you want, because it will be forgotten or because you believe you're the sole seat of God, but rather, calls us all to a broadening and opening of our field of vision into the nature of time and the very presence of God. For our dharma is not our own, not really. All dharmas are of God.

I run the yarn through my chapped hands,

Freeing it where it catches on dead skin.

Silk worms once ate green leaves and touched,

13

Small head to head, feasting,

And then cocooned themselves round in strands of light.

A spinner's hand would have drawn them anew,

And plants boiled down for the color of their skins,

Infused rainbows in the lines.

How many other lives passed over the new creation,

Labeling, measuring, boxing, shipping by air, train, ship, and car,

Displayed, inventoried,

Or simply touched, in wonder, the smooth rush of hues?

And this crochet hook,

Part of it still cries for the rocky bed in which it began,

Dug out, crushed, branded in fire, reformed, packaged, shipped,

And bought,

How many hands passing it along from stone to the shape I now hold?

And I actually have the gall to think

I make

this prayer shawl,

As I sit alone, watching the clouds

Rush by my window?

HA! And Ha!

Again.

Questions to Ponder:

1. What does the word dharma mean to you?

2. How would you explain your own personal dharma?

3. Can you think of a time in your life when you performed someone else's dharma? What were/are the ramifications of this in your own life?

4. Create a dharma mandala:

   a. On a piece of paper, create a picture or write the word for the single most important aspect of living for you. Try to be very concrete.

   b. Below this, draw or write the second most important aspect of living. Make the picture or word a part of a circle drawn around your central aspect.

   c. Continue adding circuits up to five aspects out.

   d. Now, share your mandala with others in your class. Is your life a reflection of these deep ideals? Why or why not? What would you have to do to live a life that matched your mandala?

5. How does the idea of "practicing your own dharma" apply to your work as a yoga teacher? Why is it an important idea to convey to your students?

4. Divine revelation and experience is not just given to the professional religious among us.

This idea is one of the great game changers in India's history. For millennium, spiritual power rested with the priest classes, but the Gita flies in the face of this tradition as God reveals himself in all his glory to a royal warrior. For some of us in the West, nursed on relatively liberal Protestant theology, our first response is "of course." But such nonchalance was not particularly built into India's social structure at the time.

Part of what Arjuna struggles with is the line between personal responsibility and the responsibility of others, both mortal and divine. He hasn't made the leap (in the early stages of the Gita) to his oneness with God and his fellow humans, indeed, with all creation. People still fit into roles and niches, actions are still black and white, time is still linear to him, birth and death are powerful and concrete ideas. It is interesting to watch this all begin to shift as he awakens to Krishna's teaching.

The responsibility to awaken is much more gentle than all this, though. When Arjuna *asks* Krishna to teach him, that was it! That was the small shift, the turn, even though he still felt deeply buried in his out-of-proportion sense of responsibility. Because it is not so much a throwing off of sleep but rather, a simple turn of mind to understand that there is no you-me, priest-warrior, avatar-student. They are, we are, *all one consciousness.* So of course God would be revealed to all— how could the divine not shine through, if that is the ground of all being? Monotheism, at its core, cannot be any other way. It is inevitable. For everyone!

That turn requires of us simple acquiescence: *Teach me, God.*

And the laughter that comes when you discover the truth of God
teaching him/herself is marvelous.

She rubs a little at her nose;

the trees are flowering again,

the first of the petals on the air already

wind-driven and fragrant.

The ferry blows mournful at the port,

the wild geese honk in return,

winter passing on whispering wing.

She cradles her box of sidewalk chalk

against her belly,

then presses blue to the gray concrete.

Not much traffic here in the trailer court.

And so the spring day passes,

arcs of color,

runny nose,

first daffodils nodding in her mother's

curbside garden.

"Beautiful," someone says in passing,

bound for someplace important

no doubt.

A small cat lingers on the sidewalk,

watching the play of shadow and pastel pink,

the sure movement of those small human hands,

she who hasn't learned the laws of pastel,

the boundary lines of copyright,

and the known fact that

God speaks only to

thinkers and leaders and academics and officially recognized saints;

That God must be sifted through and argued

crushed into words

that we might have

meaning.

For a moment, she looks up,

cat eyes, human eyes,

 dance

and all of creation

Recites.

Questions to Ponder:

1. What other religious traditions would agree with this idea that revelation is not just given to a special class of humanity? Be concrete.

2. How does it affect a culture if divine experience and revelation is not limited to a priest class? How does it affect an individual?

3. What sense of personal responsibility does this idea imply to you? How will it affect the way you teach Hatha Yoga?

4. Why do priest classes and professional religious exist in all cultures? What is their purpose?

5. Share what you consider to be a "religious experience." As you listen to others describe their own dances with the divine, what points seem familiar to you? Very different? Has this experience changed the way you think about "revelation" or "spiritual experiences"?

5. For the many personalities of people, there is a yoga (path to union with the divine) that is suitable for them.

One of the great strengths of the Gita is its ability to say, *no, you are not all alike in your constitutions, in the way you think, in the time and place where you have been born. Why, then, suggest that a single experiential path to God exists?* Krishna lays out for Arjuna four distinct spiritual paths, and many sub-streams, all with the intent to convey that the path to union with the divine is not singular, even though the destination is the same. Just like there is no perfect yoga pose, only the pose that is perfect for an individual practitioner, there is no one way to union with God.

The yoga of meditation (Raja Yoga), the yoga of working in the world but offering all the fruits to God (Karma Yoga), the yoga of devotion to a chosen ideal of God (Bhakti Yoga) and the yoga of deep intellectual inquiry (Jnana Yoga) are all valid and fruitful ways to dance with the divine. And indeed, in different stages of our own lives, we might find ourselves on one path for a time, then gradually merging into a new way of devotion as we mature. Just as a dance partner swirls us around, sets us in a new direction, so does the waltz with God.

This emphasis on path, you will notice, has little to do with dogma, belief, organizations or hierarchies. The Gita is a scripture about how to cultivate a personal relationship with God, and out of relationship, discover experientially that God and the seeker are not two. This is not institutional spirituality, but the very breathing heart of all religions. Buildings, priests, rites and scripture, they all pass away. In the Gita itself, Krishna says, "What use is a well when the whole world is flooded with God?" He knows that words can only point, insinuate, suggest, but only we can actually lace up our hiking boots and walk the path of our heart.

I took the bread and wine upon my tongue,

Met the eye of the minister, smiling.

Listened and sang and bowed and prayed,

And then, through coffee steam,

Leaning on elbows over a garish table cover,

I watched the congregation swirl and laugh,

Whisper, teary eyed near the bagels,

Hobble with walkers,

Walk backwards while chattering

Fuss at the chocolate all over the child's green dress.

Later, I sit on driftwood by the ocean,

Upheld by the enormous skeleton of a tree dyed

With salt and sun,

And let the wind run through me,

Chin lifted to a rare blue sky,

Eyes wide open.

If you can catch the single note in all of this,

You will have ears that hear.

KBN 2013

Question to Ponder:

1. Define and give a concrete example of a:

    a. Bhakti Yogi

    b. Jnana Yogi

    c. Raja Yogi

    d. Karma Yogi

2. If there are many paths to God, what are the ramifications for yourself or family? Your city? Your country? Your world?

3. What kind of yogi do you consider yourself to be? Why? How do you practice this path? What are its strengths? Its weaknesses?

4. Do you believe it is important for everyone to have some kind of spiritual path? Why or why not?

5. Name at one spiritual leader you respect and share why. If you were going to hang a picture of a religious leader(s) in your studio, who would it be?

6. *We have a right to our actions, but not to the fruits of our actions. These belong only to God.*

As young yoga teachers, this is one idea you should take to heart, contemplate and live from. We have a right to sit in the studio, to instruct, to nurture and support. But we are not the ones to take credit for the changes in our students. Teachers might open the door, but the student chooses to walk through and enter into the dance with the divine.

But even more than this, each time *we* sit down on the mat or meditation cushion, we do it for the sake of the action, not because it will make us stronger, more supple, more conscious of the now, or less depressed. These are what we call "fruits," and yes, they do manifest. However, if we are practicing Hatha Yoga or meditation *for* these fruits, our actions become more about ego than spirituality. It's a hard and important lesson to learn, but there is also an incredible freedom that happens when you can come to your mat or your classroom, practice uniting body-breath-mind-intuition and joy and then simply give your practice back to God. Each time you come to the mat you are new, the practice is new, and all that matters is the work itself. This is the grace we all have access to in our Hatha Yoga class.

We see this idea at play in all parts of our lives—for instance, if I write a novel to make money, to garner attention, or to please a professor, then the writing will slant that way, sullied by grabbing at the fruits rather than paying attention to the clean and pure action at hand. Both the experience of writing and the final product will suffer because I would be of two minds, one doing the work, the other focusing on what I expect/hope/fear will be the result.

So really, what we are talking about is the kind of consciousness that Arjuna, as a famous archer, was known for—perfect, one-pointed attention on the NOW. That is the very doorway to union with God.

Five dishes and a cup, totter

Messy with dried egg,

Festooned with eat utensils, cast

metal offerings around the clay-ware.

Muddy paw-prints run on the linoleum,

a ragged afterimage of morning.

Breaking Benjamin pounds out their lyrics,

and the drooping, flowerless rose shudders off

another leaf.

The cushions on the couch are damp;

spilled orange juice still drying there,

and the stack of books by the easy chair

lean

toward the bookcase, hopeful.

Cobwebs festoon the carved rafters,

three lights are out in the track,

and fog crowds up against the glass

until it ices in indecision

or liquid frustration…

Pour hot water in the sink.

Add the soap.

Reach for the first spoon,

so smooth, shimmering and light,

warmth settling into moving fingers.

Hand-crocheted washcloth dips,

grows heavy,

and so begins

the first out-breath of prayer.

Questions to Ponder:

1. When the Gita talks about "action" what does it mean? Explain.

2. How does this idea apply to your own Hatha Yoga practice?
    How does it apply to your teaching?

3. Name an event in your life when you were more concerned about
    "what you would get out of doing something" rather than the
    "doing" itself. How did this affect the action(s) you took?
    How did it affect the outcome?

4. How would you illustrate this idea to your Hatha Yoga students?

5. If you could manifest this idea continuously in your own life, what
    ramifications would it have?

7. **The sage established in wisdom is free of desires,
content, untroubled by fortune or misfortune,
free of craving, fear, anger, and aversion,
focused wholly on God.**

Sometimes, when we flip through a book of truly athletic Hatha Yoga postures or catch a beautiful pose out of the corner of our eye in class, we find that all kinds of different emotions slip through us—envy, frustration, desire, maybe even the urge to run for our coats and take up speed walking instead. This is a perfect picture of the mind cast outside of itself; the mind making us into lonely individuals who must prove, capture, overcome, push, move the world so that we are whole, protected and balanced.

As you read point seven, notice what arose in yourself—everything from a kind of poignant longing to a sense of "yeah, right, that will never, ever be me." Scripture, like a good Hatha Yoga manual, can only point to an ideal, an end result, a fruit, if you will. It is important to understand that the crafted Hatha Yoga picture, or a piece of writing for that matter, is only a touchstone. It is we who must make the journey.

This point shows us the end result of what may be many lifetimes of work on the spiritual path. The sage transcends any boundaries of dogma, religion, time and place; he or she is the figure at the pinnacle of all religions, of all spiritual paths. But to compare yourself endlessly and find yourself *lacking* is not useful. That's just another form of attachment and aversion, maybe even of anger and fear.

Instead, use this point to examine your life—where are you caught by desire? What triggers anger in you and how do you work with it? What are you afraid of? What do you run from? When does your mind slip from God? Each time you can answer such questions truthfully, and without any kind of self-loathing or self-congratulations, you take a step toward that elusive thing called wisdom.

Your first down-dog was probably shaky, dizzying, tiring. Now? You are becoming established in your down-dog, your mind and body and breath touching the ideal, but also understanding that ideals generally don't trip over the cat, drop a stone on its foot, get sick from the flu or have someone rear-end them in the parking lot. These are all things that may make the next down dog a very different experience indeed. Yet, the wisdom of the pose will continue to grow, even if the form itself is not spot-on perfect.

It is inevitable, in this spiritual tradition, that you will become the sage some day, most likely not in this lifetime, but inevitably. That very spaciousness of mind is the key, just as it is in any Hatha Yoga pose— it gives us perspective, easefulness and stability.

And that is what being a sage established in wisdom is all about.

Quiet is my practice.

Quiet upon quiet.

Too much breath, too much body, too much mind,

and

Intuition shivers alone, unheeded.

Joy?

Well, you already know—

because you, too, have sighed through the imperfect meal,

craved with sweet pain the sweater in the window,

feared the stranger's smile,

punched the wall,

cursed the bill,

danced for joy with the good news.

And when, in the closet of your heart,

you draw the prayer shawl around your shoulders,

you will see,

all the ridiculously spacious richness of your life,

where

Sitting still

Becomes

Being.

Questions to Ponder:

1. Where or when in your life have you demonstrated each of these forms of wisdom? What keeps you from being firmly established in all of them?

2. How would you explain these attributes to your Hatha Yoga class? How might you demonstrate them in your teaching?

3. Think of three people in your life or reading that you would call a sage or a person of wisdom. How can calling them to mind help you on your own spiritual path?

4. The list of the attributes of a sage might seem positively impossible to manifest. What other words of wisdom in the Gita mitigate this difficulty?

5. Is this idea of "established in wisdom" different from descriptions of religious sages in other traditions? Explain.

8. The person who thinks they kill or that they can be killed is dwelling in ignorance.

"*T*hou shall not kill!"

Yes, that is what I hear every time I read this line. And every time I get that hitch in my chest, I have to remind myself over and over that Krishna is not speaking of *relative reality* here, but rather *ultimate reality*.

There you go again, getting ready to toss the e-reader. Sit back though, and breathe a moment. Better? Then let's try to wrap our heads around this good news.

One critical point to understand as you read much of Eastern literature is that, on one hand, a clear philosophical/psychological divide seems to separate the reality we see and interact with and the reality that is the ground of all being. At the same time, relative and ultimate reality are one, but you can choose which image to bring into focus in your mind. Not one, not two, as the saying goes. Two eyes, two realities, and you can look through one at a time or both.

Let me try to illustrate this idea. You are a distinct being, with clear separation between your skin and the person sitting next to you in class. But at the same time, you breathe each other's air, the water you drink was also sipped by Jesus and Caesar. There is a reality that is larger than our individual selves, and it is singular and whole.

And the truth is, if you dig deep enough, that reality is timeless, eternal, unchanging. We participate in a constant Becoming that is both birthless and deathless. Look deeply into your own mother—she was born with the seeds of all her children within her, as was her mother, back and back into history. What does it mean to be born? It is nothing but an artificial point in time, a snapshot of the wave of all life.

And what does it mean to die? What dies? Our actions continue to ripple out, our children pass along our genetic code, the very molecules of our bodies repurposed, recycled, reused, to coin the trendy phrase. And if we were formed of dust and breath, even that is endless, the dust thrown out by the cosmos, the breath kindled by light. When you understand this reality of flesh and blood and passion and fatigue and hunger and creativity is also a single, shivering drop flung up by the ocean of the divine and then drawn back down with grace and gentleness into the vast water that is God, you begin to see through the sage's eyes.

Yes, there will come a time when, in relative reality, others will lay your body in the earth or fire. That particular manifestation of life that you cling to so mightily will appear to end. But the consciousness, the energy of NOW that ran through it continues, unabated, unstopping and forever still and present. When you can hold both—the relative body and the spirit that breathes through it, when you can see through either lens, then you'll be able to say, with Krishna, "The person who thinks they kill or that they can be killed is dwelling in ignorance."

This is *the cup that runneth over*, forever.

We dug the hole deep,

fracturing roots and

throwing up granite into the rain,

onto the slippery, muddy pile that oozed back toward its bed.

Cast like an old coat in the underbrush,

drab wool grasps at golden cedar droppings.

His hooves, once black,

Rest gray and brittle.

He flops into his grave, loose jointed at last,

his nose tucked against his chest,

his eyes, blind for years,

dull now, rusted with a long stare.

Spring will, with sharp blackberry thorns,

leap up, twisting and buoyant,

feathering out leaves that he used to eat,

and in the long shadows of fall, the vine will

open its eyes;

its own fruit,

sweet-black, reflecting light,

will fall on many tongues,

Or seed into the

bones

of the soil.

Questions to Ponder:

1. What are the moral and ethical dimensions of this teaching as you see them?

2. Why is it critical for Arjuna to understand the deeper aspect of this idea?

3. How does this statement affect your personal understanding of death and dying?

4. How might other religious traditions address this statement? How might you explain this idea to a person with a very different understanding of life and death?

5. How might you explain this idea to your students, in a language that is your own?

9. *Radical monotheism: God is both immanent and transcendent, both huge and small, both inner and outer.*

As members of a largely Christian society, we are steeped in the idea of separating the divine from ourselves, indeed, from the entire physical world. This is a system of thought called dualism, and it certainly exists in some aspects of Indian philosophy as well. As you carefully read the Gita, most of the time it feels like Krishna is very separate from Arjuna. And yet, the Yogas that Krishna is inviting us all to participate in are all about how to cross the divide from duality into union.

Emerson, Carlyle, Blake—these are just some of the names of our own "poets of the spirit" from the Romantic or Transcendental period of literature who also convey a message similar to the Bhagavad Gita, and Emerson at least had access to the Gita in the form a French translation of the work. And the powerful find at Nag Hammadi called the *Gospel of Thomas* presents what appear to be the radical monotheistic experiences of Jesus himself. So the language of this form of theology certainly runs in deep currents through our own society as well.

When you fold hands and say "namaste" at the end of a yoga class, you are embodying radical monotheism: "I greet and honor the light of God within you." The gesture is not just outwardly oriented; it is the movement of unity between yourself and another, and the recognition that at your cores, you are united.

When students begin to work with the idea that "all this is one" or phrases like "Tat Tvam Asi (Thou Art That)" confusion arises about people or objects *being* God rather than comprehending our relative world is *infused* with God or participating in God. That's where the language of poetry is helpful—we are drops gathered together in the ocean of the divine, we are all sparks of light that together create a blinding brilliance. No one of us *is the totality of* God; yet God is all of us and more.

Or as William Blake said, "see the world in a grain of sand, and eternity in an hour." Relative and ultimate reality dance together, always.

I Am the tiny bones of the inner ear,

and I Am the fog-horn, crying.

I Am the single strand of moss on the tree,

and the roots reaching and touching each other

     In darkness.

I Am the swallow's flight,

and the pilot guiding the carrier jet.

I Am the salty water drop tossed into blue skies,

and the ocean that catches it again.

I Am the festive LCD light

and the billowing super-nova.

I Am the delicate krill

and the whale who swallows it.

I Am the sand poured out of the shoe

and the desert, throwing open dry arms to the sun.

I Am the hand-spun yarn

and the loom holding me in tension.

I Am the ripe cherry

and the deer nose reaching, lipping.

I Am the warming milk on the stove,

and the soft, pink mouth of the baby,

     Opening, opening,

     an entire universe framed by delicate gums.

                        KBN 2013

Questions to Ponder:

1. How do you relate to God? Through a given form or image? As an abstract idea? Is this way of understanding and dancing with God always consistent in all situations for you? Why or why not?

2. How does the idea of radical monotheism compare to other belief systems?

3. How has your idea of the divine changed over time? What events triggered changes in your personal understanding of the divine?

4. How might this philosophy impact:

   a. Human relationships?

   b. Ecological issues?

   c. Personal psychology?

   d. Economics?

   e. A Hatha Yoga practice?

5. Does this idea impact the way you teach and respond to your students? Why or why not?

10. All living things must act; even God.

A misunderstanding often arises in spiritual practice that in order to be "holy" we have to separate ourselves out from the world. And while times of retreat are deeply beneficial to our relationship with the divine, what Krishna is pointing out is that we all are *continually* acting, even if we chose to sit in a cave with nothing but a blanket and a toothbrush. Indeed, action may be one of the very cornerstones of life. The isolated hermit still breathes, still eats and drinks, still makes an impact on the cave floor, still displaces space with his or her physicality.

And all our actions are like the actions of a dance: I adopt a dog, and that wriggling puppy instantly connects me to the breeder, its lineage, the other owners it may have had, dog food manufactures, a new carpet cleaner, and the new "doggie-doo composter" I install in my garden. Countless other ripples and permutations ripple out from that one action, not just in the physical realm, but in my mind as I worry about how to trim nails or feel the warm fur on the palm of my hand as he sleeps. My body becomes more fit as I walk him, my breath easier as I pet him, I find a poetry in his eyes, and touch joy when he races after a ball--at least on the good days!

And karma comes into play—the peace of a long walk primes me to listen to my husband's fears of work with patience and focus. The child my dog jumped up on cries out, and I see in her two-year-old eyes the beginnings of fear for things shaggy and unpredictable. Actions create reactions, both subtle and profound, energy passed through the spider web of our inter-relationship with EVERYTHING.

And the inevitability of action is what Krishna is conveying—the process, the unfolding, blending, swirling leaping up and falling back that is the larger breath of all. Our work on the spiritual path, then, is not about withdrawing—it is about finding skillful ways to move with the music of life, consciously and with joy.

Because the heart-beat called action is always there, eternally, within and without.

Time-lapse it,
1880, the island mostly barren from the loggers,
two weeks of clearing the native Rhodies and
snarl of blackberry vines,
to roll four huge logs in place,
the cabin building up on the undulating base slowly,
with thick glass and nails and wood shingled roof,
then over the years,
many feet in and out,
muddy, limping, springing, scuffing,
and the kitchen pushes into a green house,
a once-wall dissolves into a living room and
inhales a second floor,
already a hundred autumns peeling and re-peeling the paint from
old and new skin.
Mice running in the crawl space,
Banana slugs graffiti the new porch,
The cedar tree in the front yard swells,
its girth pregnant with fragrance.

Put your hand right here,

On the cracked old window frame,

And still, the echoes will vibrate your skin

The smears and washrags of lifetimes,

Caressing both today's cool rain

And the some-day fire or crack of the bulldozer,

Poised to repurpose dreams for the

Eternal Dance.

Questions to Ponder:

1. What do you think the word "action" means here?

2. If all actions create a situation of cause and effect (karma), why is Krishna demanding Arjuna to act?

3. Is meditation an action? How about daydreaming? Sleeping? Why or why not?

4. In what ways does this philosophy affirm the basic values of your culture? In what ways is it very different from those values?

5. How does the idea of action, of needing to act, affect:

    a. The idea of monotheism?

    b. Your understanding of dharma?

    c. The right to action, but not its fruits?

    d. Your role as a teacher and as a student?

Part Two:

Easing into Patanjali's

Yoga Sutras

Easing into Patanjali's Yoga Sutras

Book I: Samadhi Pada

The Portion on Contemplation

*F*or someone first approaching the *Yoga Sutras* of Patanjali without some kind of commentary, the journey can be filled with frustration. Strange Sanskrit terms that sometimes defy word-for-word translation abound, and the sayings themselves, called *sutras*, are simply a kind of skeletal frame or threads of ideas that all the complex philosophy hangs from. Add to that over 2000 years (give or take) of history, the fact that most readers are from a wildly different culture and even a different gender for that matter, and it becomes easy to toss such a difficult work to the fine-toothed combs of scholars or consign it to the status of a nifty oddity on the bookshelf.

But this need not be the case.

This small work will attempt to present *The Yoga Sutras* in a way that is more easily grasped, with exercises that will help the reader move into the world of the mind and spirit that Patanjali captured with such detail. What it will lack in scholarly footnotes and other ephemera will hopefully be made up in the presentation of a practical, useful guide to one of the truly great spiritual-philosophical work of India. And questions at the end of each chapter will encourage readers to apply what they are learning to a mat practice, since this is often the Yoga that is most familiar here in the West.

It is not meant to take the place of the Sutras themselves, only to offer an open hand on a trail that is sometimes steep and dim. Find a translation that speaks to you. Read it again and again. And return here when the going gets a little rough in spots.

So let us begin!

What in the world is Yoga?

*T*he very first sutra, in translation, says *NOW is the exposition
of yoga made.* I've capitalized the NOW because, in a sense, the entire
sutra is right here, distilled into this one bare line. Beyond meditation,
beyond *samadhi*, beyond conduct and moral and ethical concerns,
in spite of spiritual gifts and abilities, this is the very base of any yoga
practice.

OK. Maybe it is a simple statement, but we probably all agree
it is one that is much harder to practice than conceptualize. If it were
not so, Patanjali could have stopped with this first line. And indeed,
for some very adept students in Indian history, it has been enough.

I don't reckon you or I are that kind of special being, though.

Instead, Patajali unfolds the next nugget of his whole opus: he
tells us that *Yoga is a stilling of the modification of the stuff of the mind.*
In other words, yoga, which simply means "union," is that state of resting
in pure conscious awareness, where the line between the subject and
what the subject senses and responds to, and the very action of sensing
has become one. That union is the reality that our desires, aversions or
simple lethargy veil from us. Stilling the mind draws away those veils
from reality, and we are able to rest in what *is* and *what we are.*

And now Patanjali hits his stride. This first book is about the
stages of contemplation, what it is, what gets in our way, and the great
"why" of this practice. In a sense, he begins at the end, the goal, the
fruit of the practice. But then, isn't sugar often added to medicine first?

Vrittis

In this first chapter, Patanjali introduces an important Sanskrit term: *Vritti.* This word captures the whole dance of thought forms in our consciousness. Vrittis have many different forms and can be experienced in many different ways. For example:

1. They can take the form of direct perception of the world and actions there. *You see the cat walking through the shadows of a pine tree.*

2. Influence: *you notice your mother dislikes salmon and thus so do you.*

3. Scriptural belief: *you act a certain way because of what you have read or been taught in your religious upbringing.*

4. Misconceptions: when knowledge is not based in truth. *Perhaps you believe that a cold pot of water will boil faster than a warm pot (I held to this grimly as a first grader!).*

5. Verbal delusions: not understanding or interpreting what you heard incorrectly. *Remember when you used to play pass the story? One kid would whisper a long, convoluted tale in one person's ear, and then that person would tell another and so on? Then, when the original tale was revealed to the group, the ending story line sounded nothing like it.* That is an example of a verbal delusion in its grossest form.

6. Sleep: *we sometimes think that we aren't aware when we sleep, but then, how did you **know** you were sleeping?*

7. Memory: sensations, emotions and thoughts that we store that may or may not be accurate. *You remember a deer running*

through your yard, chased by three dogs almost a year ago. But later, when you relate the story to a friend, your spouse was sure there were actually four dogs.

Patanjali then tells us that we can work with all these interesting twists of our minds by practicing non-attachment to them all. To achieve *that* we engage in a practice that develops a steadiness of the mind or what we might call meditation. Again, he is saying that all of these vrittis are seen for what they are by simply being present and aware.

To make matters even more interesting, Patanjali then mentions that all these vrittis are further influenced by the basic energies of nature. He calls these basic energetic signatures *gunas,* and goes on to explain how each functions through gross physical matter. Please remember that just by being embodied, we will experience a constant shift and play of these gunas, and they can vary wildly in their strength and duration.

The first guna, *tamas*, is the energy of torpor. (Couch potato energy in other words.) Tamas can be observed when you stare at your yoga mat by the front door. And stare at it. And stare at it. It is a state of non-movement, thickness, heaviness and sloth.

The second guna, *rajas*, is the energy of action. It is the bustle of a busy kitchen, the fingers flying over the keyboard, the hawk swooping down on its prey. In its most extreme form, it can be experienced as mania and workaholic behaviors.

The third guna, *Sattva,* is the energy of balance, presence, a kind of wide- awake-and-comfortable-in-your-own-skin sort of sensation. You are neither lazy nor overzealous, neither dull nor excited. It is the still pond surface of a thriving ecosystem, the palms folded in namaste, everything still and alert. It binds us, however, because it feels so very *good*.

All three of these gunas affect how we in turn experience the vrittis. Let's say you are filled with rajasic feelings because you've had one too many cups of coffee. You look out the window and remember the time when you were a child and fell off your bike and suddenly your gut is clenching and you are on your way to the computer to write on Facebook about the need for bike safety classes for all children. That is memory under the influence of rajas. Memory was a seed, you watered it, and with the hot energy of rajas it turned into an action that could have very good or very bad consequences for you.

It's important to understand that Patanjali isn't making a value judgment about any of the gunas. They simply *are*. And the aware practitioner of yoga needs to be able to see them at play as part of being in the NOW.

Yoga is simply the stilling of the vrittis. Yoga is simply the quieting of all the stuff that ruffles the waters of your mind-body-spirit-intuition-sense of joy. Yoga is NOW.

Questions to Ponder:

Take a moment and consider how you approach your practice of Hatha Yoga.

1. Why exactly do <u>you</u> practice?

2. What is the state of your mind in various poses? Compare a warrior pose to a child's pose. What did you learn about your body, your breath, your mind, your intuition, and your sense of joy?

3. How does the breath create a bridge between the mind and body? How does the texture of the breath echo the state of your mind? Your body?

4. Do any of the vrittis surface on your mat? How do you work with them? How could you help your students understand these phenomena?

5. Are you aware of the play of the gunas within your practice? Explain.

What is Samadhi?

As we continue our exploration of the first book of Patanjali's Yoga Sutras, we come next to the discussion concerning the different stages of samadhi. *Samadhi* is one of those lovely Sanskrit terms that defy an easy translation into English. Often, it is equated with meditation, but the way Patanjali uses this word is much closer to a state rather than a practice. For our uses, samadhi is **the state cultivated by the practice of meditation**. This, for Patanjali, is actually the true starting point of the path of Yoga.

First he speaks of *samprajnata samadhi* (distinguishing samadhi) and says it is characterized by the presence of reasoning, reflecting, rejoicing and a sense of I-am-ness. Notice the progressively finer and more subtle apprehension of self-consciousness as he breaks this term down into the following categories:

1. *savitarka samadhi*= focus on very gross objects. From within, you deeply understand the physical properties of a seashell on your altar.

2. *savichara samadhi*=your focus deepens to the constituent elements of the shell, the smallest and most subtle elements that create all of matter called the *tanmatras* in Sanskrit.

3. *sa-ananda samadhi*=the blissful awareness of simple and pure consciousness that you share with the shell, that underlies even the subtle elements of matter.

4. *sa-asmita samadhi*= you begin to hold only the barest thread that you are experiencing the shell. The wholeness of the shell and yourself begins to blur into a single point.

Finally, as the practice deepens, the yoga reaches a state of *asamprajnata samadhi*: the "I" sense disappears, the ego released. There is no difference between the reality of the shell and yourself, between your neighbor and yourself. It is all one consciousness. This is the birth of the *jivamukta*, the person who is alive but liberated, who walks in the full light of realization yet keeps a material body. Patanjali says this samadhi arrives through the vehicles of faith, strength, memory, contemplation-meditation and discernment (being able to distinguish the real from the unreal).

Patanjali understands that the purpose of meditation is to still the mind to allow these various kinds of samadhi's to unfold Without the basic ability to hold the mind steady on a gross object, the rest is much harder to realize. It is also the stillness of the mind that allows us to move from an intellectualization of the states of samadhi to an experience of them. This is very important to understand, because as you read this it may all make perfect sense, but when you try to experience these levels of samadhi, you will often find that they slip away from your grasp like mist. The good news of the *Yoga Sutras* is that eventually everyone will realize their true nature and awaken. Nobody gets left behind, ever, even if it takes thousands of lifetimes to wake up. There is no denying reality; the real will "out" in the end.

When Patanjali speaks of faith, its important to understand that he is not advocating one particular deity or one particular religion. Yoga is not a religion per se; it is an experience, a life-path that transcends all dogma and institutionalization. But in all that intellectualization, Patanjali is quite adamant about *devotion*.

But devotion to what? The term the writer of the Yoga Sutras uses is *Ishvara Pranidhanat*, or your chosen ideal. For Patanjali, this means a supreme consciousness, omniscient and unconditioned by time. Notice this definition resonates with the idea of the Godhead in Christianity, of Allah in Islam, the Great Spirit of many Native American tribes, the Tao of Lao Tzu. Patanjali will later show that this supreme consciousness can be visualized in any gross form or understood as something that sustains the very ground of our existence. As many people who practice yoga, there are that many faces of God.

In the yogic tradition of India, there is a lovely phrase: *Ekam sat, vipraha bahudha vadanti*: *Truth is one, seers express it in different ways.* Imagine if the entire world were able to really digest this one saying, to deeply understand that the impulse to turn to the divine inevitably takes on the colors and flavors of a given culture and time, yet are all beautiful expressions of that one, timeless, omniscient consciousness. Each religion and face of God sits like a bead upon a thread that runs through them all. Love your neighbor as yourself because your neighbor *is* yourself. Love other religions because they, too, shine with the light of Ishvara.

Time for a special note to the Teachers and Students of Hatha Yoga:

Sometimes new students of Hatha Yoga think the physical practice of asana is the kind of Yoga that Patanjali is speaking of. And when they start to read, they immediately ask questions like, "Where are the postures, the breath work, the Om jewelry and all the paraphernalia like mats and blocks and straps of the modern world?" The answer is simply that Hatha Yoga was one among many different ways to realize union in ancient India, and not a very popular one at that. The Yoga Sutras are not about Hatha Yoga at all, although much of the wisdom in the writings can be *applied to* a modern practice.

Originally, Hatha Yoga was considered an incredibly difficult and ascetical practice, with strict and rather uncomfortable guidelines to bring the body under the subjugation of the mind and will and then, from that point, to begin to transcend them both. It was a practice designed by men for men and really tough men at that. In fact, it largely died out in native India until brought back into the beginnings of popularity after India's independence.

What we call Hatha Yoga in the United States is really often nothing more than a kind of sport or at its worse a way to lose weight and look good in $100 designer clothing. This Olympic season, I shuddered when I again heard rumors of instituting Hatha Yoga as an Olympic sport. It would no more belong there than "Olympic Rosary Telling" or "Olympic Lectio Divina." I also recently read an email from a woman who "had burned off over 300 calories" in her flow-yoga class, as if this was the very be-all and end-all of the path. Truthfully, such folks would be better off in an aerobics class (burns more calories), weight lifting (fights osteoporosis more effectively) or going for a walk (less stress and cost of getting to a class).

But at its best, the West has really done a lovely job of reinterpreting the rigorousness of the practices and essential disdain for the limitation of the physical body that characterized classical Hatha Yoga into an art-form that unfolds the poses from the inside out, that cultivates the attitude of ahimsa (non-harming) from within one's own self, that transcends gender and even physical liabilities into the very ground of a spiritual path. So while writing as a scholar of comparative religion, I would say we are not practicing "traditional Hatha Yoga" in the United States. Thank God. As a nearly life-long practitioner of Yoga, I am deeply thankful and excited that it is being interpreted in new and sophisticated ways by women and men, and for all ages and physical abilities of people. In that sense, Hatha Yoga in the West is keeping the tradition green and organic and alive.

Questions to Ponder:

1. When we say that Hatha Yoga is a tool, a prayer practice, *how* do you bring your own religious orientation to the mat? Is it in the form of an intention, an offering of the practice back to your understanding of the divine? Explain.

2. What ideal of God do you hold? In other words, how do you name the mystery to yourself? Krishna, Jesus, Allah, etc? How does your practice of Hatha Yoga inform and interact with this ideal?

3. Create your own examples of the different levels of samadhi as you understand them now. Put them someplace where you can find them each year. As part of your New Year's celebrating, pull them out and see if your understanding, if your examples, have changed with time.

4. How would you, as a yoga instructor, make space for all religions and concepts of the divine in your class? How would you respond to someone that says they cannot practice Hatha Yoga because they feel it is a different religion?

5. In your own words, how does the practice of Hatha Yoga prepare one to experience the different states of samadhi? Or could you argue that the intention of Hatha Yoga is something very different? Explain.

Book II: Sadhana Pada

About Practice

But Really, Why Practice if we are already THAT?

*N*ow, for most new yoga students, we sort of hit a little wall here. Yea, we can see the gunas and vrittis at play in our own minds. Yea, we are intrigued with all the different stages of samadhi, maybe even intrigued by the idea that we can realize our seamless unity with the divine. But is there any practical reason why we should be inclining our ear to Patanjali? Is there a breathing, useful point to all of this?

The answer is, yes!

Patanjali writes, "*To one of discrimination, everything is painful indeed, due to its consequences: anxiety and fear over losing what is gained; the resulting impressions left in the mind to create renewed cravings; and the constant conflict among the three gunas which control the mind*" (Satchitananda, Trans., p. 100).

OK, now you are saying, "Whoa! Everything is painful?" I bet you are lining up your blessings, the graces of dark chocolate and coffee, the walks in the spring woods, the lover who has just kissed your cheek, and you are getting ready to really fight the idea that everything is "painful indeed." The word that Patanjali uses, though, to indicate "pain" is actually the Sanskrit term *duhkha* which might better be translated as "unsatisfactory."

Even that might have you tapping your foot and frowning right now. But lets tease this apart a bit. Lets say there is a lovely sweater on sale in the nice shop down the street. You save for a couple weeks to buy the sweater, forgoing fresh veggies and eating spagettios so you can finally bring it home and yes, it is lovely, a pleasure to wear. But then you begin to fear having it on while you eat your spaghettios. Or wearing it when you visit a friend who has a cat that sheds clumps of hair as a vocation. In these instances, you are experiencing kinds of pain. First, the craving of wanting the sweater was a kind of pain. Then the getting it and keeping it perfect is a kind of pain, and finally after it has sat in your closet for a year, you'll start noticing other sweaters, and craving them, and yes, that is a kind of pain as well. The getting of the first sweater didn't stop the craving for the new and improved. Now you can see why perhaps unsatisfactory is a better translation—there is nowhere in this cycle to just be, *to rest* in a place that isn't craving and isn't avoiding. As you begin to really look at your experiences, you'll see this pattern generating itself over and over.

And then you remember: **Yoga is the stilling of the thought-waves of the mind.** And desire, pain, attachment, aversion, these are *all* thought waves. How would you feel if you craved nothing? Avoided nothing? Maybe, if you are honest, you might feel free, relaxed, even a little expansive and full. But is that even possible?

Yea! ***"Pain that has not yet come is avoidable"*** (Satchitananda trans, 101). That's great news! There is a way to put a little hitch in the wheel of revolving attachment and aversion! For Patanjali, the way is realizing the conflating of the True Self (*Purusha*) and that all this mess, glorious and fun and playful as it sometimes can be (*Prakriti*), is at its base inaccurate. We identify ourselves with our sweaters and our jobs, our roles and relationships. But we are not those things. And how do we tease ourselves out of that net? Well, that "how" is what the second portion of the Yoga Sutras are all about.

Questions to Ponder:

1. Try to think of something you really want and walk yourself through the feelings that arise around that object or person. Are they steady and eternal, or do they fluctuate and morph over time?

2. Identify the places in your heart/mind where you crave something or avoid something. List them so you can see them. Are *you* these things? What will they actually bring to you or take from you? Is there something within you that is greater than these things? What is that?

3. Ask yourself over and over again, "Who am I?" Try to shoot for at least 25 answers to this question. Are any one of them *really* you? So "who" are you?

4. How does a personal ideal of the divine help with the process of resting in that place that is neither attached nor avoiding the play of matter around you?

5. How does your Hatha Yoga practice shed light on this idea of duhkha, and on spirit (Purusha) and nature (Prakriti)?

Ashtanga Yoga

The First Limb:

Yama: The Actions that Lead to Suffering

We are now entering the section of the text that covers the path called Ashtanga Yoga (Eight-Limbed Yoga). In a sense, this is where Patanjali begins to drop down from lofty states and ideas into the very heart of *practice*. Notice this is not the Hatha Yoga practice called Ashtanga Yoga—it is the path to union with the divine as set out by Patanjali over 2000 years ago. And yes, if you have studied Buddhism, you will most likely have an 'ah-ha' moment coming! (For fun, try comparing Patanjali's Yoga to the Buddhist Eight-Fold Path; there you will find both a profound resonance and very stark differences.)

The yamas, the first limb of this yoga, include: not causing pain, not lying, not stealing, not wasting the gift of your sexuality or practices of purity, and not coveting. These are not commandments, however! Each of the yamas point to the different ways we both suffer and cause suffering in the world. And suffering *creates* waves in the mind, which then draw the possibility of quiet meditation and union away from us. No divine entity will trigger the pain; you do so yourself because of the very nature of this world.

The entire structure of ashtanga yoga is like the warp on a loom—lines of tension and direction through which we guide the weft of our actions and experiences to create a pleasing, strong and brilliant fabric.

As you work through each of the yamas below, keep in mind that their manifestations can be subtle or gross, and contain many hues and textures.

Not Causing Pain *(ahimsa):* On the gross level, this could mean not killing, not doing physical violence. On the subtle level, this could mean not gossiping, or even thinking ill of a person or situation. Thought is action, remember. (Already, you may get an inkling about how profoundly hard it is to practice this yoga; why lifetimes might be required to "get it." It is important, as with all meditation paths, to not use the path itself to beat yourself up. "I failed at this!" is just another form of causing pain. Hold the ideas lightly, but firmly and choose to live out *the experiment* of walking more softly and gently in the world.)

Not Lying (*satya***):** On the most obvious level, this means trying to speak the truth or remain silent when the truth might be harmful to voice. At a more inward level, this means not hiding reality from yourself, not thinking out of the paradigm of the lie.

Not Stealing *(asteya):* The heaviest form of this warning is to not take what does not belong to you in the physical environment. But it can also be about not taking the energy or space of expression from another living thing.

Not Wasting the Gifts of being embodied (*brahmacharya*):
Often this means to live a "pure" life with all your being, not squandering the energies of life in ways that are not directed to God. If you are married, it means being true to your mate. In the more subtle sense, can mean things like "not lusting in your heart" for those things that would cause suffering.

Not Being Greedy (*aparigraha*): The hues of greed can range from constant and obvious coveting of people and things, or the more deeply entrenched values of a holding onto our time just for ourselves and trying to live out of a sense of hoarding.

As you read the yamas, notice how they tend to come in groups when you experience life. Make up a fictional story for yourself that shows how each of the yamas can come into play, each building and sustaining the others. Remember, we are working more with the idea of creating a fabric of life here, rather than a list of punitive dos and don'ts. The yamas and niyamas hold us, rather than bind us.

Questions to Ponder:

1. What other religions capture all or part of these moral teachings? Is there any difference in the *intent* behind such teachings? Explain.

2. Use a concrete example from your own life to illustrate the idea of dukkha (the unsatisfactory nature of material life).

3. Create a picture for yourself that captures all five yamas, using colors and images that arise from your own experiences.

4. How have you observed these yamas in your own Hatha Yoga practice? How will you choose to work with them in future? Be concrete.

5. One way to work with the yamas and niyamas is to create your own rule of life, a set of simple actions you hold to as you go about your work and play and rest. For instance, perhaps you will add to your "rule of life" the practice of not talking about someone unless they are present. Or maybe you will choose to abstain from buying something new for at least three days after the impulse for it has arisen. Begin now to create a rule of life for yourself, one that will speak directly to the work you need to undertake with yourself.

The Second Limb:

Niyamas: Actions to Cultivate in the World

Niyama could be translated as actions and states to cultivate to decrease suffering. They include purity, contentment, discipline, study of spiritual texts, and the worship and devotion to your understanding of the divine. Again, like the yamas, there are gross and subtle manifestations within you of each of these.

Purity (*saucha*): Purity can range from following strict dietary and environment rules to opting to avoid the yamas deep in your own thoughts. Jesus taught this best when he said that we are not defiled by what we put into our mouths, but rather, by what comes out of them.

Contentment (*samtosha*): If one simple rule truly sums up all the yamas and niyama, it would be this word. Contentment soothes greed, lust, anger, the need to cause pain. It makes practicing purity of the mind easy even as it fuels a gentle and unhurried inquiry into the divine's nature. It is the very heartbeat of all the Yogas.

Discipline (*tapas*): The word tapas is usually associated with the creation of heat, to simmer as it were, all the elements of a yogic practice. It can take the form of your Hatha Yoga practice as you develop the fire and determination of daily practice, or it can be a deep inner vow to awaken, much like the idea of the inner jihad of Islam or the state of mind Arjuna finally reaches on the battlefield under Krishna's tutelage.

Study of spiritual texts (*svadyaya*): In the Christian monastic tradition, the monks understood that merely reading a religious text is not the same as developing a relationship with it. The words must be taken down into the deepest corners of the mind and heart and then given life in our own actions. Otherwise, they are just objects on our shelves. Chant in many religious traditions is often used to facilitate this, and with good reason. Often seniors who are largely non-communicative are still able to sing songs from their youth. Music stores within us not just *information*, but *emotive energy* in a way that is easily accessed. Words also give us a kind of focus, a sense of another present with us as we walk our path. They are the fabric of human relationship and so spending time with our "written" spiritual friends supports us deeply on the journey.

Devotion to your understanding of the Divine (*Isvarapranidana*): This element of the niyamas might mean the overt practice of worship and prayer offered to your understanding of Reality, but it can also mean the constant offering of all your actions, all your thoughts, all your self to God. In the Christian tradition we come across the phrase "to pray without ceasing." In Buddhism, the state of mindfulness in all areas of life is cultivated so the practitioner is in constant interaction with reality as it is NOW. Like the words of scripture that are taken in deeply, devotion to reality calls you into relationship, even to the point of unity (union, yoga).

The niyamas, then, are what help mitigate the tendency to drift into the less skillful actions of the yamas. Comforted and enlightened by scripture, seasoned in contentment, and supported by a relationship with the divine, purity and discipline are delightful, joy-filled and spacious.

Questions to Ponder:

1. What do you consider to be your most treasured spiritual texts? How did these texts come to hold the place in your life that they do? Explain.

2. How do you express your devotion to your understanding of the divine? In what ways could you use your Hatha Yoga practice to deepen this sense of devotion?

3. How do you define discipline? Apply the idea of the three gunas to your definition. Is your understanding of discipline balanced and non-harmful? Explain.

4. What niyamas could you add to your personal "rule of life" in a way that speaks directly to your own needs at this time? How would you work with them creatively?

5. How do you think the yamas and niyama contribute/distract from the process of awakening? Go through both lists and create concrete example for yourself where you can see these elements at play in your own life.

The Third Limb: Asana

A quick flip through the Yoga Sutras will show you that there isn't a single Hatha Yoga pose mentioned. The word asana (posture) here points to taking the meditative seat, which should be easeful and stable. And yet, these two hallmarks of the body grounded in the present moment are remarkable companions to invite into your Hatha Yoga practice as well.

When you are in any pose, take a moment to notice: are you stable? Are you easeful? I often call up an image of Quan Yin seated in her "royal posture," one knee bent, one leg draped long, one arm resting on her bent knee, one arm strong by her side, her spine erect. There is nothing sloppy or unfocused about it, yet she is the picture of perfect ease. Out of the very stability of her mind, her body rests in ease. All possibilities inherent in both action and stillness have become one. This is the ultimate posture of union that can also act.

The yogic system of life on this earth rests on five koshas or "levels of embodiment." They include the body of food (the physical self), the body of breath, the body of our mind, the body of wisdom and intuition and the body of joy. Each level is progressively more subtle but each level stirs and reflects the others; pluck one "string" of this system and the whole vibrates. Patanjali here is setting up the food body, by making it stable and easeful, to transmit its message of focus and attention to the other levels of the embodied meditator. The tall, stable, easeful seat slows and supports the breath. The stabilized breath in turn allows the mind to become still and luminous. The stabilized mind opens us to wisdom and intuition, and resting with ease and support in that state frees joy to vibrate back up through the system.

A quick word about joy—it is not a happy-happy, throwing confetti up in the air kind of energy. It is more like Julian of Norwich's famous line, "And all shall be well, and all shall be well, and all manner of things shall be well." It is blue-sky mind, wide open, spacious, a great Yes to all things within and without, the vast affirmative that is our deepest response to life.

Questions to Ponder:

1. Draw a picture or write a poem that expresses the idea of "joy" for you.

2. Play with several different meditative positions—sitting in a chair, kneeling, sitting cross-legged, laying down. What are the pros and cons of each posture? How does the mind/body react to each style of "seat"?

3. What objects can you identify in nature that illustrate the twin ideas of stability and easefulness. Could you bring a photo or example into your classroom or practice space to remind you of these qualities?

4. What keeps you from being easeful or stable in your meditative posture? How do you work with these energies and sensations?

5. Sometimes we are instructed not to move in our meditative posture. What do you think Patanjali would say about this? What do you personally think about this?

The Fourth Limb

Pranayama: Cultivation of the Breath

*H*ave you ever wondered why working with the breath through counting, retention, observation and so on holds such an important place in nearly all the great religions of the world? For some, the breath is equated with spirit, the very presence of God within and around us. In other traditions, the breath is the vehicle for the life force, the energizing principle that shifts gross matter into something full of movement and joy. For yet others, the breath is our most constant companion, the link between the conscious controlling mind and the largely unconscious processes of the body. As companion, it becomes an object of meditation that is always at hand. We have already explored, too, how calming the breath calms the entire embodied system—physical self, mind, intuitive self and joy all enter into union on the wings of a calm, deep breath.

Notice the progression that Patanjali has laid out so far: by becoming aware of the actions that cause us suffering and the actions that mitigate that suffering (yama and niyama), we are better able to take the meditative seat with poise and calm, ease and stability (asana). And out of this base, the breath can be viewed and worked with in an attitude of relaxed clarity. The fabric of the yogi is starting to grow more complex and yet also more unified. From the actions of life to sitting still, from sitting still to working with the more subtle energies of the breath, we are being drawn "down and in" toward union with God.

Yet subtle does not mean weaker or less important. There is an old story in India where the various operations of the body were vying for who was the most powerful. One by one, they left the physical body, and yes, being without vision, or hearing or taste was uncomfortable, but when breath left for just a few minutes, everything within the body ceased, all movement, all perceiving, all thought. And all the aspects of the body bowed deeply to the breath—to the animating energy of the divine that calls us forth from the clay.

Questions to Ponder:

1. Put on a piece of rock and roll music, and really enter into the spirit of the rhythm. As the song draws to a close, notice the rate and depth of your breath. Now put on something soft and gentle-- an adagio or soft chant. Again, check in with your breathing. How do you think your other senses influence the way you breathe?

2. Focus your eyes on one small object—maybe a clock face in your studio, or the nap of your yoga mat. After a minute, notice the nature of your breath. And then broaden your gaze, soften your eyes and use your peripheral vision. Again, after a minute, observe your breath. How were the two experiences different? What impact would focused or diffuse awareness have on your yoga practice?

3. What breath-work would you add to your "rule of life"? Why?

4. How would you explain to a beginning yoga student why breathing throughout the practice is so important? Can you make your explanation concrete and easily demonstrated? How?

5. Try this: Tighten up as many muscle groups as you can, and then chant the word OM or another word or phrase that has meaning to you. Now, utterly relax and chant the sound again. What are the differences between the two experiences?

The Fifth Limb

Pratyahara: Pulling away from the Senses

When I was a young teen, I remember watching a movie about a military robot that had been struck by lightening and had "awakened" as a truly sentient creature. Like a young child, he raced around, hollering for input, input, input—tastes, sights, sounds, textures, ideas. He was insatiable. And only after a period of time, after processing all that input in relationship with humans, was he capable of two enormous acts: he was able to see himself as part of the divine dance of life and he was able to *laugh*.

We are not so very different from that robot come to life and if we are very lucky, we too will learn that we are more than our input and be able to laugh joyfully with it all. Pratyhara, the fifth limb of Ashtanga Yoga, calls us to move away from our senses consciously and willingly. It is the movement of down and in, the slowing of input into our ever-hungry minds, a chance to experience that something really exists below the level of senses, and that something is consciousness.

This is the stage of preparing the mind for a different kind of relationship, one where all our points of reference are released, a groundlessness that is a kind of surrender, an attitude of all the senses being at rest that is the best state for a deeper kind of listening, seeing, smelling, tasting and touching. It is the posture of pure acceptance, full of the same ease and stability hinted at in the meditation asana. We learn that we are not our senses, and that clarity folds another thread into the cloth of our Yoga.

Questions to Ponder:

1. Can you think of other meditative systems that ask you to move away from your senses? Where in the Christian Bible is this hinted at?

2. Define pratyahara for a new yoga student, using your own concrete examples to illustrate and clarify your words.

3. Where does the exercise of humor come in handy in your meditative practice? On your mat?

4. Sometimes, this experience of withdrawing from the senses will tend to bring up deeply buried memories, random thoughts, etc. Looking back at the yamas and niyamas, can you see hints of how to work with these energies? How do you know when a student might need the support of other psychological professionals in your area? How would you broach such a subject with them (or with yourself!)?

5. How do you think periods of sense withdrawal might impact the times when your senses are very active? Give concrete examples in your explanation.

The Sixth Limb

Dharana: Concentration

*D*harana, or one-pointed concentration blooms out of the deep surrender of all the senses. Because our minds are no longer being pulled this way and that by sensation, our minds begin to focus naturally. The attitude of surrender gives way to a kind of refined steadiness that is both incredibly narrow and incredibly wide at the same time. Freed from the tyranny of the constant input, bringing our minds to heel from mental ripples like memory, thought, and strong emotions, the station of dharana is like focusing on a single note from a flute, letting it both touch us and fill the void around us. We begin to become that single note.

There is still a sense of will here; just as the ego's will surrendered the senses, the will is employed yet again to hold attention steady, like a candle flame in a breathless room. It is working with the energy behind the act of seeing, smelling, tasting, touching, and hearing. Having no senses to flow out into, that energy become more powerfully directed inward.

It is like this: imagine if you could stand in your living room when it is ablaze with television and conversation and the scent of your dinner, then started to turn things off one by one, allowing even the more subtle stimuli to gently fade until you stood with just a single candle in your hand. The whole world would both narrow to that single point of light and yet you would also feel the entire womb of the living room holding you, each sensation enfolding and supporting the other. And then you closed your eyes and that rift between perfect focus and perfect openness narrows. That is the very experience of dharana.

Questions to Ponder:

1. Where do you use deep focus in your daily activities? What is its function? How does it differ from how Patanjali is using the idea of focus in his yoga?

2. Can you differentiate between a focus that is tight and willful, and a soft holding sensation of focus? Try working with a single object—a flower or candle flame. Hold the image with your eyes open, and then close your eyes and hold the image. Can you identify why your mind may not be able create a one-pointed attention on the object? Each time it varies, open your eyes and begin again. Notice any tendency toward aggression or aversion as you work with the practice.

3. Is there a difference between the idea of focus and attention? Explain.

4. Draw a picture or write a poem about how you experience a focused mind.

5. Can you ever experience dharana in a Hatha Yoga practice? Why or why not?

The Seventh Limb

Dhyana: Meditation

*H*ere the yogi has only a breath of ego tied to the experience. Body has settled to become easeful and stable, the breath stills and nearly disappears from conscious awareness, the senses are all at rest, the mind focused and broad at the same time (what we might call the internal face of present moment awareness). Now the state of meditation exists, the perfect abiding with only the barest sensation of "I am experiencing this."

The struggle, though, has softened, the fierce determination and heat of all the other limbs cooling into deepest stability and easefulness. And even the gentle inkling that this is a kind of grace, a return to our most basic state, held by God, is no longer important or substantial.

Release that last finger of ego. And grow vast.

Questions to Ponder:

1. What single word can you think of that captures the energy of meditation as you understand it? Or can you find another way to illustrate it?

2. There are many different kinds of techniques that call themselves "meditation." How do these differ from how Patanjali uses the term here?

3. In what ways do you think "meditation" might be different from savasana (the "relaxation" or "corpse" pose in modern parlance)?

4. How would you explain the difference between concentration and meditation?

5. Looking back up at the progression of Patanjali's treatment of ashtanga yoga can you create a picture that illustrates how the "fabric" of the practice is knit together?

The Eighth Limb

Samadhi: Absorption

And then it happens, the first taste of non-duality that you recognize only because you fall back into meditation, into the recognition of ease and stability and being held by God.
In samadhi, the "I" becomes absorbed in the totality that is God. Words begin to fail, because there are no points of reference, only the hints of the experience arise when you return to even a subtly dualistic state.

I have always loved the Christian "philosophical poem" that goes:

Be still and know that I am God.

Be still and know that I Am.

Be still and know.

Be still.

Be.

(And then, in Samadhi, the perfect silence after the "Be," the perfect reunion, signals the end of duality.)

Questions to Ponder:

1. What keeps you from entering into this state in your practice? Be concrete.

2. Our culture tends to be very wary of "navel gazing." What does Patanjali's Yoga offer the material world? What gifts do you think it brings to yourself and others?

3. Compare the progression of Patanjali's Ashtanga Yoga to your own prayer practices or meditation practices. What is different? What is similar?

4. What is the difference between the practice of a spiritual path and "holding beliefs"?

5. How would you explain the difference between meditation and samadhi in a way that is easy to grasp?

Book III: Vibhuti Pada

The Portion on Accomplishments

*I*n this section of the Yoga Sutras, Patanjali examines the *siddhis*—the extraordinary gifts that come with the practice of yoga. But the chapter is as much a kind of warning. Yes, this and that will happen. And what does it all mean?

In terms of your path to awaken, they don't mean a thing.

In a sense, many of the siddhis are potentially lovely hooks that threaten to reinvest you in the energies of wanting and avoiding. They stand as markers that something is happening to "you," but can only be used wisely when there is no "you" there to make use of them. In a sense, they are like charismas of Christianity, gifts and skills that are rooted firmly in God and not the individual ego, yet do manifest in matter.

Patanjali includes the following:

1. You understand not just the physical flow of the evolutionary process, but also the energy that works through it all.

2. By hearing the sound of any word, even one from a different language, the meaning becomes clear. You sense the meaning in the vibration of the word.

3. You remember your past lives accurately and with discrimination.

4. You are able to read the bodies of others, and through this subtle observation, know their thoughts, but not the motive behind the thoughts.

5. You become invisible to others.

6. You are able to know the time of your own death.

7. You are able to transmit friendliness and other positive qualities to others.

8. You are able to access the very strength of nature.

9. You are able to see into the very foundations of matter (energy).

10. You are able to deeply understand the cosmos and beyond.

11. You gain mastery over hunger and thirst.

12. You experience visions of masters and adepts from all ages.

13. You deeply understand the relationship between the physical world (relative reality) and the non-dual underpinnings of it all (ultimate reality).

14. You experience spontaneous intuitive gifts and super-sensitive senses.

15. You can mentally stand within another's body.

16. You can leave the body at will and bend the "laws" of physics.

17. You glow with a kind of light.

18. You acquire the ability to become very small, very big, very light, very heavy, achieve all your desires, create anything and command and control everything.

19. You naturally radiate a physical beauty.

And so on...

Certainly as you gaze on this list, you might compare it to the accomplishments of our great spiritual masters like Jesus or Buddha. But then, for the spiritual aspirant, comes this warning:

"By **non-attachment** even to that (all these siddhis), the seed of bondage is destroyed and thus follows Kaivalya (independence)" (Pada III: 51). In other words, the point is not the "powers" here but your ability to let go of even these remarkable states and charisms. Because Patanjali says, essentially, these are the products of the focused mind. They can snare you again, because you fall into the trap of "I do this or that." Only when "the tranquil mind attains purity equal to that of the Self, there is Absoluteness" (Pada III: 56).

Questions to Ponder:

1. Why do you think these siddhis begin to manifest in yogis and saints of other traditions? What is their use?

2. Why might these siddhis impede the process of awakening?

3. Have you ever experienced any of these siddhis in your life? Observed them in others?

4. Do you think a person can be awakened and not overtly show any of these abilities?

5. As you look over the list, can you come up with subtle and gross examples for each? (In other words, if we say a "light surrounds a person," how might this manifest? As a physical glow? As a sense of health and vitality? As a feeling that, through interactions with their world, people themselves feel more clear and vibrant?)

Book IV: Kaivalya Pada

The Portion on Absoluteness

*I*n this final book, Patanjali lays out the deep philosophical underpinnings of his entire yoga and the fruits of practice. Let's take a quick look at his most important ideas:

1. **Fully awakened souls function spontaneously with grace; they are not driven by the willful ego or by past karma.**

   The fully awakened person still acts, but he or she is not being driven by the gunas, nor the energies of attachment and aversion. There is a sense that the force of God works directly through the person, and so each action performed comes from a deeper source. The awakened person has become the true instrument of the divine—still at play in maya, but not ensnared by it. Past karma is also withdrawn as the energy or impulse behind action, and the awakened person does not create any fresh karma to work through.

2. **Body and mind are material; the soul is pure consciousness. "Soul awareness does not evolve from matter. Soul awareness enlivens matter and expresses itself through material form." (Davis, 208)**

There is a saying in India that without "Shakti, Siva is a corpse." This captures the spirit of this second idea—that matter is animated from within, and that the soul or atman is primary, matter a secondary covering through which expression, education and other actions occur. Take matter away, and consciousness remains—it is unaffected by the transformations of constituent parts. And that consciousness is what you are!

3. **We tend to see the whole object before us rather than the constituent parts, or the energy beneath these.**

We easily can identify a tree in our yard. But when we look deeper, we begin to see water, earth, sky, as well as the chemical processes that breathe the tree into life. And even deeper than the constituent parts of the tree, we must look very close indeed to catch the raw energy that is the base for the smaller parts that make up the object we call a tree. No wonder that teachers like Vivekananda and Yogananda both pointed directly at the language of science when teaching; like a scientist, we are called to look deeply into matter and come face to face with the divine.

4. **Mind orders, stores and mixes the impulses of the senses, but the atman is the seat of gnosis. In other words, the mind serves the soul.**

The mind can record and store, mix and generate material from its experiences, but this is not the same as "knowing" in the deepest sense. When we are awakened, we see even the play of mind as a servant to the abiding consciousness we call the divine. We no longer confuse our true Self with the ever-fluctuating elements of matter.

5. **The very desire to be liberated is necessary to attain awakening; to transcend even this desire requires grace.**

It's fascinating that when you begin to look at the play of desire and aversion in your life, their role as educators becomes very clear. Yogis hit an interesting point in their lives, though: the energy to awaken is a kind of desire. So how do you drop this impulse to move into gnosis? The answer Patanjali gives is that "you" are not the one to transcend it at all—the gnosis of the divine, once awakened, nullifies the karmic energy of the desire. You no longer *desire* to awaken because you *are* wakefulness or pure consciousness itself.

Questions to Ponder:

1. How can *you* tell the difference between actions that are driven by the gunas and karma and actions of a realized saint?

2. Compare this idea with other religion's understanding of the nature of soul and matter and the Divine. How is it the same? How is it different? Does this idea change the way you see your Hatha Yoga practice? Why?

3. Why might "seeing the constituent parts" of matter be important? What hint does it give us about the nature of Reality?

4. What is the purpose of our minds according to what you have learned about Patanjali's Yoga?

5. Grace is a tricky word. What does it mean to you? How would it really apply to Patanjali's philosophy and description of practice?

A final thought—

*A*ny exposition on the thought of another, especially flavored with the biases of translators and our time and place in history, is a sobering thing at best. I end, then, with my favorite reminder to all who move toward the deepest states of knowing, including (and even especially) myself:

I who know, and do not know that I know:

Let me be whole

Let me be awake.

I who have known, but do not know:

Let me once more see

The beginning of it all.

I who do not wish to know,

But still say that I wish to know:

Let me be guided

To safety and light.

I who do not know,

And know that I do not know:

Let me, through this knowledge, know.

I who do not know, but think that I know:

Set me free

From the confusion

Of that ignorance.

(Anonymous Islamic Prayer)

Blessings on your journey!

Kimberly Beyer-Nelson, fellow seeker and companion in God

Works Cited

Davis, Roy Eugene. *Life Surrendered in God: The Kriya Yoga Way of Soul Liberation.* CSA Press, Lakemont, GA. 1995.

Hawley, Jack. *The Bhagavad Gita; A Walkthrough for Westerners.* New World Library, Novato, CA. 2001.

Satchidananda, Sri Swami. *The Yoga Sutras of Patanjali.* Integral Yoga Publications, Yogaville, VA. 2008.

www.ingramcontent.com/pod-product-compliance
Lightning Source LLC
LaVergne TN
LVHW021130190326
834317LV00008B/251